How to Address Hormonal Imbalance

Women's Health Solutions

Dani Raymond

Table of Content

Introduction

A. The Significance of Hormonal Imbalance in the Health of Women

The issue of hormonal imbalance in women's health is very important. Hormones are essential for controlling a wide range of biological activities. An imbalance in these hormones can have a significant effect on a woman's general health and well-being

We will examine the role that hormone imbalances have in women's health, going over the causes, signs, and possible outcomes of these imbalances along with various management and therapy choices.

Several factors can contribute to hormonal imbalances in women:

A hormonal imbalance occurs when the body's regular hormone levels and interactions are disturbed. Hormones such as estrogen, progesterone, and testosterone are crucial for controlling mood, fertility, menstrual cycles, and numerous other physiological functions in women.

These imbalances can happen at various stages of a woman's life, from puberty to menopause.

Causes of Hormonal imbalance:

Hormonal imbalances in women can be caused by a number of circumstances, including:

1. Puberty: A woman's life undergoes major hormonal changes as she reaches puberty. Mood fluctuations and irregular menstrual periods may result from the oscillation of estrogen and progesterone levels.

2. Menstrual Cycle: The entire menstrual cycle is marked by hormonal changes. This equilibrium can be upset by diseases like polycystic ovarian syndrome (PCOS), which can result in irregular menstruation and problems with fertility.

3. Pregnancy: As the body adjusts to accommodate the developing fetus,

hormonal imbalances are frequently experienced throughout pregnancy. Mood swings and morning sickness are two symptoms that might result from these abnormalities.

4. Menopause: With a drop in progesterone and estrogen, menopause is a major hormonal shift. Symptoms like mood swings, heat flashes, and a decrease in bone density may arise from this.

5. Stress: Prolonged stress can cause abnormalities in the body's cortisol and other stress hormone levels. Menstrual cycles, fertility, and general health may all be impacted by this.

6. Diet and Lifestyle: Hormonal equilibrium can be upset by poor diet

and bad lifestyle decisions like smoking or binge drinking.

7. Medical diseases: Hormonal imbalances can also result from some medical diseases, such as diabetes and thyroid issues.

8. Medicine and Birth Control: Hormone levels can be impacted by both hormonal birth control and medicine. Imbalances may occur in certain women when these treatments are started or stopped.

Symptoms of Hormonal Imbalance

A woman may experience a different symptom than another due to hormonal abnormalities. Typical symptoms consist of:

1. Irregular Menstrual Cycles: Variations in the duration and pattern of monthly cycles.

2. Mood Swings: Anxiety, despair, and mood swings can all be caused by hormonal changes.

3. Weight Gain: Hormonal imbalances, such as those caused by insulin and thyroid hormones, can result in weight gain.

4. Fatigue: A decrease in hormone levels may cause weariness and a low energy level.

5. Hot Flashes: During the menopause, hot flashes are frequent and unexpected feelings of heat that are frequently accompanied by perspiration and a flushed face.

6. Insomnia: Sleep patterns can be disturbed by hormonal changes, which can result in insomnia.

7. Acne and Skin Issues: Dryness and acne are two conditions that can be brought on by hormonal abnormalities.

8. Hair Loss: Hair thinning or loss may be brought on by changes in hormone levels.

9. Changes in Libido: Sexual function and desire can be impacted by hormonal abnormalities.

The effects of an unbalanced hormone

A woman's health might suffer greatly from hormonal abnormalities. These imbalances may have an impact on one's emotional, psychological, and physical health. Among the possible outcomes are the following:

1. Infertility: Some women find it difficult to conceive as a result of hormonal abnormalities, such as PCOS or thyroid conditions.

2. Osteoporosis: Reduced bone density due to low estrogen levels during and

after menopause increases the risk of osteoporosis and fractures.

3. Cardiovascular function: Imbalances in hormones, particularly in the menopause, can affect heart function and raise the chance of developing heart disease.

4. Emotional Health: Hormonal imbalances can cause mood swings, despair, and anxiety, which can have an impact on a woman's emotional health.

5. Sexual Health: A person's general quality of life and close relationships may be strained by changes in libido and sexual function.

Managing and Treating Hormonal Disproportion

The underlying reason and the intensity of symptoms determine how hormone imbalances in women's health are managed and treated. Several popular strategies consist of:

1. Lifestyle Changes: Hormone regulation can be achieved by leading a healthy lifestyle that includes stress reduction, regular exercise, a balanced diet, and frequent exercise.

2. Medication: To relieve menopausal symptoms, hormone replacement therapy (HRT) is frequently utilized. Certain hormonal abnormalities may require the prescription of additional drugs.

3. Surgery: To treat conditions like endometriosis or uterine fibroids, surgery may be advised in certain circumstances.

4. Dietary Modifications: Particularly in cases like PCOS, dietary modifications including cutting back on sugar and processed foods might help balance hormones.

5. Counseling and Therapy: Managing the emotional and mental effects of hormone abnormalities might be helped by psychological support.

6. Alternative Therapies: To assist control hormones and reduce symptoms, some women look into complementary therapies including

yoga, herbal supplements, and acupuncture.

In summary, an important aspect of women's health is hormonal imbalance. A woman may experience these imbalances at different points in her life, which can result in a variety of symptoms and possible negative outcomes. In order to address these imbalances and enhance general well-being, it is imperative to comprehend the causes, symptoms, and possible remedies.

In order to receive appropriate counsel and help in controlling hormonal imbalances and maintaining their health, women should seek advice from healthcare specialists.

Chapter 1: Understanding Hormonal Imbalance

A. Definition of Hormones and Their Function in the Body

Hormones are vital chemical messengers that are crucial to the way the human body operates. They are secreted into the bloodstream by different glands and serve to regulate and govern a multitude of physiological functions. In-depth discussions of hormones' properties, functions, and vital roles in preserving homeostasis and general health will be provided in this piece.

The Meaning and Types of Hormones

The endocrine system's specialized glands and cells create hormones, which are organic substances. Hormones that are released by these glands into the bloodstream can reach specific cells or organs all across the body. The pituitary, thyroid, adrenal, and pancreatic glands are among the glands that make up the endocrine system. These glands are responsible for secreting different hormones.

There are various categories of hormones, such as:

1. Steroid Hormones: These include cortisol, aldosterone, and sex hormones (testosterone, progesterone,

and estrogen). They are generated from cholesterol. Usually, they affect target cells gradually.

2. Peptide hormones: These include oxytocin, growth hormone, insulin, and other hormones made of amino acids. They often take effect rapidly and fade soon.

3. Amino Acid-Derived Hormones: These are produced by the adrenal glands and include norepinephrine and epinephrine, sometimes known as adrenaline.

4. Serotonin, dopamine, and melatonin are examples of monoamine hormones, which are a subclass of hormones generated from amino acids.

Control of Hormones and Feedback Loops

Feedback systems carefully govern hormone release and regulation in order to preserve homeostasis. The body releases or inhibits certain hormones in response to changes in a certain parameter, such as blood glucose levels, in order to restore those levels to their ideal range.

For example, the pancreas secretes insulin to increase glucose absorption into cells, which lowers blood glucose levels when blood sugar levels rise after a meal. On the other hand, when blood sugar levels fall, the liver releases stored glucose into the bloodstream as a result of the pancreas' production of glucagon.

Stable blood sugar levels are maintained in part by this feedback loop.

Major Hormones and Their Functions

1. The pancreas secretes insulin, which controls blood sugar levels by encouraging the absorption of glucose into cells for energy or storage as glycogen in the muscles and liver.

2. Thyroid hormones (T3 and T4): The thyroid gland produces these hormones, which are essential for controlling body temperature, metabolism, and energy expenditure.

3. The adrenal glands secrete the chemicals adrenaline and

noradrenaline, which prime the body for the "fight or flight" response. In stressful situations, they dilate airways, elevate heart rate, and release stored energy.

4. Cortisol: Another hormone produced by the adrenal glands, cortisol plays a role in how the body reacts to stress. It aids in blood pressure maintenance, inflammation suppression, and metabolic regulation.

5. Growth hormone (GH): The pituitary gland secretes this hormone, which encourages cell division and growth. It is essential for childhood growth and aids in the maintenance of tissues and organs in adulthood.

6. Estrogen and Progesterone: These two sex hormones control the menstrual cycle, secondary sexual traits, and pregnancy. They are produced in lower amounts by the testes in males and by the ovaries in females.

7. Testosterone: Mainly generated in the ovaries of females and the testes of males, testosterone is important for the development of secondary sexual traits in males as well as for the maintenance of bone density, muscular mass, and general health in both sexes.

Hormones' Significance to the Body

Hormones are essential for many processes and functions within the body. Their effects on growth and development, mood, energy levels, and immune responses are just a few of the many functions they play.

The following are some other facets of hormone function:

1. Reproductive Health: In order to regulate the menstrual cycle, ovulation, and pregnancy, hormones such as estrogen, progesterone, and testosterone are critical.

2. Bone Health: Growth hormones and estrogen play a major role in preserving the strength and density of bones. Osteoporosis and other

disorders may result from a decrease in these hormones.

3. Emotional Well-Being: The regulation of mood is greatly influenced by hormones, especially dopamine and serotonin. Anxiety and depression are two mood disorders that can be exacerbated by imbalances.

4. The thyroid hormones play a major role in controlling body temperature. Disorders like hyperthyroidism or hypothyroidism can result from such imbalance.

5. Regulation of Metabolism and Weight: Hormones such as ghrelin and leptin affect appetite and hunger, and thyroid hormones control metabolism.

Weight gain or loss may be attributed to hormonal abnormalities.

6. Immune Function: The immune system is modulated by several hormones, such as cortisol. The immunological response might be weakened by prolonged stress and high cortisol levels.

Health issues and Hormonal Imbalances

Multiple different health problems might occur from hormonal abnormalities. Typical instances includes:

1. Diabetes: Type 1 or type 2 diabetes can be brought on by inadequate

insulin production or insulin resistance, which raises blood sugar levels.

2. Thyroid Conditions: A variety of symptoms, including disruptions in metabolism, can result from hypothyroidism (an underactive thyroid) or hyperthyroidism (an overactive thyroid).

3. Menstrual irregularities: Polycystic ovarian syndrome (PCOS), irregular menstrual periods, and other reproductive health problems can result from hormonal abnormalities in women.

4. Hormone-Dependent malignancies: Sex hormones have an impact on certain malignancies, including

prostate and breast cancer. One common kind of treatment is hormone therapy.

5. Osteoporosis: Women are more likely to develop osteoporosis due to bone loss brought on by a drop in estrogen following menopause.

6. Mood Disorders: Depression and anxiety are examples of mood disorders that can be exacerbated by hormonal abnormalities, namely those involving serotonin and dopamine.

Hormone Replacement Therapy

Medical therapies such as hormone replacement therapy (HRT) may be administered in cases of hormonal imbalances or shortages. In order to restore hormonal balance, hormone replacement therapy (HRT) uses synthetic or bioidentical hormones. Men with hypogonadism and women going through menopause are two common examples of replacement therapy.

However, due to possible side effects and related health hazards, HRT is not without risk and should be carefully studied and monitored under the supervision of a healthcare practitioner.

Hormones are the unsung heroes of the human body, regulating a myriad of functions vital to overall health and wellness. Our bodies depend on their delicate balance to function at their best, and any disturbance in this balance can result in a number of health problems.

Maintaining general health requires an understanding of the functions of hormones and the significance of hormonal balance. It's critical to speak with a healthcare provider if you believe you may have a hormonal imbalance since they can accurately diagnose the condition and suggest the best course of action for reestablishing balance in the body's complex endocrine system.

A. Typical Reasons for Hormonal Unbalance

Hormonal imbalances can impact people of all ages and genders and can arise for a number of causes. Hormonal imbalances have a number of common causes, including:

1. Stress: Prolonged stress can raise cortisol levels, which over time can throw other hormones out of balance in the body. Numerous health problems, including weight gain, sleep difficulties, and psychological disorders, may arise from this.

2. Poor Diet: Hormonal imbalances may be caused by a diet heavy in processed foods, sweets, and unhealthy fats. For example, eating too much sugar can cause insulin resistance, and unhealthy fats can

influence the hormones that are produced, such as testosterone and estrogen.

3. Absence of Physical Activity: A sedentary lifestyle can affect the balance of hormones involved in metabolism and blood sugar management, resulting in weight gain and insulin resistance.

4. Medical diseases: The endocrine system may be disturbed by a number of medical diseases. For instance, women with PCOS may experience imbalances in their sex hormones, while thyroid conditions may impact the levels of thyroid hormones.

5. drugs: A few drugs have the potential to affect the production or

function of hormones. This covers several antipsychotic medications, corticosteroids, and birth control pills.

6. Menopause and Aging: Natural hormonal changes can result from both menopause in women and aging in both genders. Men may have decreasing testosterone levels after menopause, but women usually have a reduction in progesterone and estrogen during this time.

7. Estrogen, progesterone, and thyroid hormones are just a few of the many hormones that can fluctuate significantly throughout pregnancy and the postpartum period.

8. Environmental Toxins: Hormone function can be disrupted by exposure

to environmental toxins, such as pesticides, pollutants, and endocrine-disrupting compounds found in some plastics.

9. Abuse of Substances and Alcohol Excessively: Certain recreational substances and alcohol can upset the hormonal balance, especially in the liver and pancreas.

10. Sleep Deprivation: Not getting enough sleep can cause hormonal imbalances that affect metabolism, energy levels, and general health. These hormones include growth hormone and cortisol.

11. Obesity: Excess body fat, particularly around the abdomen, can upset the balance of sex hormones and

cause insulin resistance. The hormones that control hunger and body weight, ghrelin and leptin, may also be impacted.

12. Thyroid Disorders: Issues with the thyroid gland can lead to disorders including hypothyroidism and hyperthyroidism, which throw off the body's normal thyroid hormone balance.

13. Autoimmune illnesses: Autoimmune illnesses, which include type 1 diabetes and Hashimoto's thyroiditis, are caused by the body's immune system attacking its own tissues, which can result in hormonal abnormalities.

14. Genetic Factors: Some people may be more prone to diabetes, thyroid issues, or hormonal malignancies due to a genetic predisposition to specific hormonal imbalances.

15. Tumors: Hormone synthesis can be disrupted and hormonal abnormalities can result from benign or malignant tumors in the endocrine glands. An excess of adrenal hormones, such as cortisol, may result from an adrenal tumor, for instance.

It's crucial to remember that, depending on the particular hormones involved, hormonal imbalances can present with a broad range of symptoms and health problems. Changes in weight, mood fluctuations, abnormal menstrual cycles, exhaustion, and other symptoms are possible. It's critical to see a healthcare provider if you think you may have a hormone imbalance for a diagnosis and recommended course of action.

D. Identifying Signs and Symptoms

For an early diagnosis and course of therapy, identifying the symptoms and indicators of hormonal imbalances might be essential. The specific hormones involved determine how these abnormalities present themselves. The following are some typical indications and symptoms of hormone imbalances:

1. Irregular Menstrual Cycles: Women may experience irregular, heavy, or

painful periods, which can be indicative of hormonal difficulties, such as polycystic ovarian syndrome (PCOS) or thyroid diseases.

2. Unexplained Weight Changes: Thyroid dysfunction, insulin resistance, or other hormonal imbalances may be the cause of sudden weight gain or reduction without dietary or exercise modifications.

3. Weariness: Hormone abnormalities such as those involving the thyroid, cortisol, or insulin may be the cause of chronic weariness and low energy.

4. Mood swings: Anxiety, despair, impatience, and mood swings can all result from hormonal abnormalities.

These could be linked to abnormalities in neurotransmitters or variations in sex hormones.

5. Skin problems and acne: Variations in sex hormones, especially before or during pregnancy, can cause acne. Insulin and cortisol abnormalities can also cause skin problems.

6. Hair Loss: Thyroid hormone or sex hormone abnormalities may be linked to alopecia, or thinning hair.

7. Libido Changes: Unbalances in sex hormones, such as low testosterone in men or low estrogen in women, can be associated with a drop in sex drive.

8. Hormonal imbalances can cause digestive problems, such as diarrhea,

constipation, or bloating. These problems are frequently linked to illnesses like irritable bowel syndrome (IBS).

9. Sleep disturbances: Unbalances in melatonin, cortisol, or other chemicals that regulate sleep can lead to insomnia or disturbed sleep patterns.

10. Hot Flashes: Among women, hot flashes may indicate the onset of menopause, which is marked by altered hormone levels and a reduction in estrogen.

11. Excessive Sweating: Hyperthyroidism and other hormonal abnormalities can cause excessive perspiration or night sweats.

12. Increased Thirst and Frequent Urination: Hormonal disorders like diabetes or abnormalities in the antidiuretic hormone (ADH) may be linked to increased thirst and frequent urination.

13. Infertility: Problems with reproduction and fertility can be attributed to hormonal imbalances, especially in women with PCOS or males with low testosterone.

14. Breast Changes: Thyroid or sex hormone abnormalities may be linked to breast lumps, discomfort, or size changes.

15. Bone Health: Sex hormone abnormalities, especially in

postmenopausal women, can lead to a reduction in bone density or fractures.

16. Cardiovascular Symptoms: Adrenal hormone imbalances, such as those involving aldosterone or adrenaline, can be linked to high blood pressure, palpitations, and irregular heart beats.

17. Modifications in Appetite: Hormonal abnormalities can impact signals of hunger and satiety, which may result in modifications to one's appetite and eating habits.

18. Headaches: Especially in women during their menstrual cycle, hormonal migraines are frequently associated with changes in sex hormones.

19. Skin Pigmentation: Variations in skin pigmentation, such as hyperpigmentation, or darkening of the skin, may indicate diseases linked to hormones, such as Addison's disease.

20. Cold Sensitivity or Intolerance: In hypothyroidism, in particular, intolerance to cold temperatures may be linked to thyroid hormone abnormalities.

It is noteworthy that although these indications and symptoms may suggest hormonal dysregulation, they are not exclusive to any one ailment. They may also be the consequence of other health problems. It's critical to see a healthcare provider for a comprehensive assessment, diagnosis, and suitable therapy or management if you have severe or persistent symptoms. Medications and lifestyle modifications can frequently effectively treat hormonal abnormalities.

Chapter 2: Hormone Imbalance Diagnosis

A. Medical Assessment and Examination

It's crucial to have a medical assessment and tests to identify the underlying cause if you think you may have a hormone imbalance or if you are exhibiting symptoms and indicators that may be connected to hormonal problems. What to anticipate along the process is as follows:

1. Consultation with a Healthcare Professional: Depending on your gender and particular symptoms,

make an appointment with a primary care physician, endocrinologist, gynecologist, or urologist. They will ask about your symptoms, obtain your medical history, and do a physical examination.

2. Blood Tests: The most popular and reliable method for determining hormone levels is blood testing. To measure the levels of hormones in your bloodstream, your healthcare practitioner may request particular blood tests based on your symptoms and any suspected hormonal imbalances.

Typical hormone testing consists of:

- Thyroid Function Tests: To evaluate thyroid function, these tests examine thyroid hormone (T3, T4) and thyroid-stimulating hormone (TSH) levels.

- Sex hormone tests: Based on your symptoms, these tests may examine your levels of progesterone, estrogen, testosterone, luteinizing hormone (LH), and follicle-stimulating hormone (FSH).

- Cortisol Tests: If you have symptoms associated with stress or adrenal function, these tests can evaluate your cortisol levels and diurnal cortisol rhythm.

- Insulin and Blood Glucose Tests: These tests assess blood glucose levels and insulin sensitivity, which are critical in situations when diabetes or insulin resistance may be suspected.

- Pituitary Hormone Tests: These examinations evaluate the hormones, including prolactin and growth hormone, that are secreted by the pituitary gland.

3. Imaging examinations: When there is a suspicion of tumors or anatomical problems, imaging examinations such as CT, MRI, or ultrasounds may be utilized to assess the anatomy of the endocrine glands.

4. Tests for Stimulation or Suppression: In these tests, particular chemicals are given to induce or inhibit the production of particular

hormones. To assess insulin resistance, for instance, the oral glucose tolerance test is employed.

5. Tests on Urine: Urine samples taken over the course of a day can be used to assess various hormones, including cortisol and certain catecholamines.

6. Saliva Tests: When determining the diurnal regularity of cortisol release, saliva tests are a useful tool for measuring cortisol levels.

7. Genetic Testing: To find particular genetic mutations that can cause hormone imbalances, genetic testing may be necessary in some circumstances. This is especially important in cases of congenital

adrenal hyperplasia and similar disorders.

8. Thyroid Ultrasonography: This imaging modality can be used to assess the anatomy of the thyroid gland and identify any anomalies, such as nodules.

9. Bone Density Testing: A dual-energy X-ray absorptiometry (DXA) scan may be carried out to test bone density in cases of suspected osteoporosis or problems with the health of the bones.

Your symptoms and the hormones that are suspected of being out of balance will determine which tests and examinations you specifically need to go through. It's critical that you heed the advice of your healthcare physician and voice any worries or inquiries you may have throughout the assessment procedure.

The underlying cause of the hormone imbalance will determine the therapeutic options available after a diagnosis has been determined. In situations of tumors or structural anomalies, treatment options may include hormone replacement therapy, medication, lifestyle modifications, or surgery.

It's critical to schedule routine check-ups with your healthcare practitioner in order to assess your progress and modify your treatment plan as needed.

B. Getting Expert Assistance

Getting professional assistance for any health issues, including imbalances caused by hormones, is an essential part of taking care of your wellbeing.

Here's a how-to guide for obtaining professional help:

1. Identify Your Symptoms: It's critical to identify and note your symptoms before seeking assistance. Your healthcare professional will find this information useful during the assessment procedure.

2. Select the Correct Healthcare Provider: You should consult a general practitioner or a specialist initially, depending on your unique symptoms

and concerns. Endocrinologists, or hormone specialists, gynecologists, or urologists, or even psychiatrists or psychologists, if mood-related symptoms are a concern, are common experts for hormonal disorders.

3. Make an Appointment: Get in touch with the office of the healthcare practitioner of your choice to make an appointment. Start with a general practitioner if you're not sure which kind of specialist to see; they can send you to one if needed.

4. A record of your symptoms, any pertinent medical history, and a list of any current prescriptions or dietary supplements should be brought to your consultation. Having these data at hand will facilitate an accurate

diagnosis by your healthcare professional.

5. Ask Questions: Don't be afraid to clarify anything and ask questions throughout your appointment. You might want to find more about recommended tests and evaluations, possible courses of therapy, and anticipated results.

6. Tests and Evaluation: To determine the underlying reason of your hormone abnormalities, your healthcare provider may suggest blood tests, imaging investigations, or other diagnostic procedures based on your symptoms.

7. After a diagnosis has been made, heed the advice of your healthcare

practitioner regarding your course of treatment. This could involve medication, hormone replacement treatment, lifestyle modifications, or other therapies. Make sure you follow the prescribed course of action and show up on time for any follow-up appointments.

8. Be an Advocate for Yourself: Do not be afraid to get a second opinion from a different healthcare professional if you believe that your issues are not being sufficiently addressed or if your treatment plan is not working.

9. Keep Lines of Communication Open: Communicate with your healthcare practitioner on a frequent basis. Throughout your therapy, let your doctor know if your symptoms

change, if you have any adverse effects, or if you have any concerns.

10 Lifestyle Modifications: To assist your treatment, you may need to make modifications to your lifestyle, depending on the diagnosis. These could involve adjustments to your nutrition, exercise regimen, and techniques for handling stress.

11. Assistance and Resources: Take into account obtaining assistance from associations, discussion boards, or support groups associated with your particular ailment. Making connections with people who have gone through comparable experiences can offer insightful knowledge and emotional support.

Recall that getting expert assistance is a proactive move toward enhancing your well-being and standard of living. In many cases, hormonal imbalances can be successfully controlled or treated under the supervision of a skilled medical professional. Find the best treatment plan that suits your needs by being patient with the procedure, which may take some time.

Chapter 3: Hormonal Health and Lifestyle Factors

A. Food and Hydration

Hormonal balance and general health are significantly influenced by nutrition and diet. Your body's ability to produce and regulate hormones is influenced by the food you eat. Some essential factors for a diet that is hormone-friendly and well-balanced are as follows:

1. Optimal Macronutrient Balance:

- Lean protein sources such as fish, poultry, legumes, tofu, and lean meat cuts should be included in your diet.

For the synthesis of hormones and general health, protein is necessary.

- Carbohydrates: Select complex carbs from foods like fruits, vegetables, and whole grains. Steer clear of processed foods and high amounts of refined sugar as these might cause insulin abnormalities and blood sugar increases.

- Healthy Fats: Include fats from nuts, seeds, avocados, and olive oil, among other sources. The synthesis and operation of hormones depend on these lipids.

2. Rich in Nutrients Foods:

- Fruits and Vegetables: Packed with antioxidants, vitamins, and minerals, these foods promote general health. Zinc, vitamin C, and D are a few nutrients that are very crucial for maintaining hormone balance.

- Fiber: Eating a diet rich in fiber can help control insulin and blood sugar levels. Additionally, it promotes digestive health, which has an indirect impact on hormone balance.

- Omega-3 Fatty Acids: Rich in flaxseeds, walnuts, and fatty fish (such as salmon and sardines), omega-3 fatty acids offer anti-inflammatory and hormonally-supportive qualities.

3. Hormone-Friendly Options:

- Phytoestrogens: Foods high in phytoestrogens, such as legumes, flaxseeds, and soy products, can balance the body's estrogen levels.

- Iodine: By supplying enough iodine, seafood, seaweed, and iodized salt can support thyroid function.

- Selenium: Foods high in selenium, such as brown rice, sunflower seeds, and Brazil nuts, can help maintain thyroid function.

- Antioxidants: Consuming foods high in antioxidants, such as berries, dark leafy greens, and vibrant veggies, can help shield cells from harm and promote general well being.

4. Sufficient Hydration:

Maintaining adequate hydration is crucial for good health and may also have a secondary effect on hormone balance. Numerous physiological functions, including the movement of hormones via the bloodstream, depend on water.

5. Control of Portion:

- Gaining weight as a result of overeating might exacerbate hormone abnormalities. Be careful of portion sizes and engage in mindful eating.

6. When to Have Meals:

- Consuming many meals and snacks throughout the day can help control blood sugar levels and avoid hormone surges and crashes.

7. Cut Back on Added Sugars and Processed Foods:

- Additive sugars and bad fats found in highly processed foods can throw off hormonal balance and cause weight gain.

8. Resolve Stress:

- Hormone imbalances connected to stress, such as cortisol, might result from prolonged stress. Take up stress-relieving activities like yoga, deep breathing, meditation, or frequent exercise.

9. Steer clear of excessive caffeine and alcohol:

- Hormone function and sleep patterns might be affected by excessive alcohol and caffeine consumption. Drink these drinks in moderation.

10. Personalized Method:

Remember that every person has different nutritional needs. It is best to speak with a qualified dietitian or nutritionist if you have a specific hormonal condition. They can offer you individualized advice and food plans that are catered to your requirements.

In addition to being important for overall health, eating a nutritious, well-balanced diet can help maintain hormonal balance. However, for individualized advice on how nutrition might help you achieve your health objectives or if you have suspicions about a particular hormonal problem, speak with a healthcare professional or a qualified dietitian.

B. Working out and Being Active

Physical activity and exercise are essential parts of a healthy lifestyle and have a big impact on hormone balance and general wellbeing. Frequent exercise has several advantages, one of which is how it affects the body's hormones. This is how exercise affects hormone balance and explains why it's so important:

1. Insulin Regulation:

- Exercise increases insulin sensitivity, which facilitates cells' better utilization of glucose. Insulin imbalances are the hallmark of illnesses like type 2 diabetes and insulin resistance, which can be prevented and managed using this approach.

2. Control of Cortisol:

- Exercise, especially cardiovascular exercises like swimming or jogging, can lower cortisol levels and aid in stress management. Hormonal imbalances and a host of health problems are linked to prolonged stress and high cortisol levels.

3. Production of Growth Hormones:

- Growth hormones are released in response to specific types of exercise, such as strength training and high-intensity interval training (HIIT). This hormone is essential for the development, maintenance, and repair of tissues.

4. Thyroid Activity:

Frequent exercise can help maintain a healthy thyroid, which is necessary for proper hormone balance and metabolism. It can be especially helpful for those who are hypothyroid.

5. Endorphin Production:

- Endorphins, which are organic "feel-good" hormones, are released when you exercise. These hormones have the power to elevate mood and lessen depressive and anxious symptoms.

6. Estrogen Equilibrium:

- Exercise can help women's estrogen levels stay balanced. For women who are getting close to menopause, when estrogen levels may drop, this can be especially crucial.

7. Regulation of Testosterone:

- Men's healthy testosterone levels are crucial for maintaining muscle mass and general health. Resistance training and vigorous exercise can help men maintain these levels.

8. Maintaining Weight:

- Regular exercise helps maintain a healthy weight, which can significantly affect the balance of hormones. Hormone abnormalities related to insulin, estrogen, and other substances can result from excess body fat, particularly in the abdominal area.

9. Enhanced Sleep:

- Sleep patterns improved by physical activity have been shown to positively impact hormonal balance, including melatonin and cortisol regulation.

10. Bone Wellness:

- Weight-bearing activities, such as jogging, weight training, and walking, can increase bone density and lower the chance of osteoporosis, a condition that is impacted by hormone fluctuations.

11. Heart-Related Health:

Frequent exercise lowers the risk of heart disease and associated hormone imbalances, supporting cardiovascular health.

12. Menstrual Well-being:

- Women who exercise can experience a reduction in symptoms related to hormone imbalances and help maintain normal menstrual periods.

13. Mental Health:

Exercise can enhance memory and cognitive function, which are impacted by hormones such as brain-derived neurotrophic factor (BDNF).

14. Immune System:

Frequent, moderate-intensity exercise helps strengthen the body's defenses against infections by boosting the immune system's performance.

15. Blood Pressure Management:

- Blood pressure can be regulated by exercise, which lowers the chance of hormonal imbalances linked to hypertension.

It's crucial to remember that different types, lengths, and intensities of exercise can affect hormone balance in different ways. Finding a fitness regimen that you enjoy and can stick with over time is crucial. Before beginning a new fitness regimen, always get medical advice, especially if you have any underlying medical issues.

Including regular exercise in your daily regimen is a proactive way to maintain hormonal balance and advance general health. Finding the ideal balance for your body and lifestyle is crucial, whether it be through yoga, weight training, cardio, or other types of exercise.

C. Stress Reduction

For hormone balance and general well-being to be maintained, stress management must be effective. Hormone imbalances caused by prolonged stress, such as those involving cortisol, can have a major effect on your health. The following are some methods for stress management:

1. Physical Activity: One of the best strategies to lower stress is to exercise regularly. It encourages the release of endorphins, which naturally elevate mood. Aim for at least 75 minutes of strenuous activity or 150 minutes of moderate-intensity aerobic activity each week.

2. Mindfulness & Meditation: Engaging in deep breathing exercises or mindfulness meditation might help you de-stress. Additionally, these

methods can aid in reducing cortisol levels.

3. Yoga: To encourage relaxation and lower stress levels, yoga incorporates physical postures, breathing techniques, and meditation. It can enhance general wellbeing and assist with hormone balance.

4. Progressive Muscle Relaxation: To relieve physical strain and stress, this technique entails tensing and then releasing various muscle groups.

5. Sufficient Sleep: Make sure you get enough good sleep, since hormone balance and stress recovery depend on it. Try to get seven to nine hours each night.

6. Balanced Diet: Consume a range of foods high in nutrients as part of a balanced diet. Stress can be caused by nutritional imbalances, so give whole grains, lean meats, fruits, and vegetables first priority.

7. Limit Alcohol and coffee: Consuming too much alcohol or coffee can make stress and sleep problems worse. Lower your consumption if required.

8. Social Support: Continue to communicate with loved ones. Stress can be reduced and emotional support can be obtained by talking to a trustworthy person.

9. Time management: Set priorities for your responsibilities and organize your

work. Feelings of overwhelm can be lessened with good time management.

10. Establish Realistic Goals: Be honest with yourself about your capacity for success each day or week. Stress can arise from having unrealistic expectations.

11. Relaxation Methods: Examine methods for relaxing such as aromatherapy, taking warm baths, or relaxing to calming music.

12. Journaling: Maintaining a journal can assist you in identifying stressors and in exploring your feelings and responses to them.

13. Limit Screen Time: Especially before bed, cut back on your exposure

to stressful material like social media and the news. Sleep quality might be impacted by screen time.

14. Professional Assistance: If you're finding it difficult to control your stress on your own, you might want to think about getting help from a therapist, counselor, or mental health specialist.

15. Interests and Leisure Activities: Taking part in interesting interests and activities might help you de-stress and relieve stress.

16. Don't overcommit yourself; instead, learn to say no. Saying no to further obligations when your plate is already full is acceptable.

17. Achieve a good balance between your personal life, career, and self-care. It's critical to prioritize self-care and avoid letting work-related stress rule your life.

18. Reframe your perspective on pressures in order to improve your mindset. Occasionally, you can lessen the tension that a situation causes by altering your perspective on it.

Recall that learning how to effectively manage stress is an individual process. One person's ideal solution might not be suitable for another. Try out various tactics to determine which one(s) best suits your needs for stress management. Your general health and well-being can be enhanced and hormonal balance can be supported by lowering stress and encouraging relaxation.

D. Hormone Reactions to Sleep

Sleep is essential for maintaining hormonal equilibrium and general wellness. The length and quality of sleep have a direct impact on the body's hormonal systems. Here's how hormones are affected by sleep:

1. Cortisol Control:

- The body's main stress hormone, cortisol, is closely regulated in relation to sleep. A healthy diurnal cortisol rhythm is maintained by getting enough restorative sleep. Prolonged sleep deprivation raises cortisol levels, which are linked to stress and can throw off the hormonal balance.

2. Production of Growth Hormones:

- Rapid eye movement (REM) sleep and deep, slow-wave sleep (Stages 3 and 4 of the sleep cycle) are when most growth hormone (GH) is secreted. Growth hormone (GH) is required for tissue upkeep, repair, and growth. Decreased GH production may result from poor sleep.

3. Sensitivity to Insulin:

- The control of insulin sensitivity and blood sugar levels depends on sleep. Lack of sleep can reduce insulin sensitivity, which can cause abnormalities in insulin and blood sugar levels. Type 2 diabetes and insulin resistance are at risk due to this.

4. Regulation of Ghrelin and Leptin:

Hormones that control hunger, including ghrelin and leptin, are influenced by sleep. Lack of sleep can cause an increase in ghrelin, a hormone that stimulates appetite, and a decrease in leptin, a hormone that suppresses it. Metabolic imbalances and weight gain may result from this.

5. Thyroid Substances:

- Sleep affects thyroid hormones, which control metabolism. Sleep disorders, especially insomnia, can throw off the body's thyroid hormone balance.

6. Girls' hormones:

- Maintaining a normal secretion of sex hormones, such as testosterone and estrogen, requires getting enough sleep. Sleep issues can cause these hormones to become disrupted, which can impact reproductive and sexual health.

7. Creation of Melatonin:

- The body receives a signal to rest via the secretion of the sleep hormone melatonin during dark hours. Melatonin production can be disrupted by changes in sleep habits and exposure to artificial light at night.

8. Regulation of Appetite and Weight:

Lack of sleep can cause abnormalities in the hormones leptin, ghrelin, cortisol, and insulin, which are all linked to hunger, satiety, and metabolism. Obesity and weight increase can be attributed to these abnormalities.

9. Stress Hormones and Mood:

- Sleep has a direct impact on stress reduction and mood control. Stress hormone imbalances, including cortisol and adrenaline, can result from sleep deprivation.

10. Immune System:

- Sleep is necessary for the immune system to operate correctly. Sleep deprivation can impair immunity and make a person more vulnerable to diseases.

11. Cognitive Function and Memory:

- Sleep is essential for cognitive function and memory consolidation. Sleep quality has an impact on hormones that are involved in these processes, such as brain-derived neurotrophic factor (BDNF).

It's critical to emphasize excellent sleep hygiene and make sure you consistently get enough high-quality sleep in order to support hormonal balance and general wellness. Most grownups need seven to nine hours of sleep every night. Here are a few pointers to enhance your sleep:

- Adhere to a regular sleep schedule by setting aside time each day to go to bed and wake up.
- Establish a cozy and tranquil sleeping space.
Restrict your time spent using screens and artificial lighting before rest.
Steer clear of caffeine and stimulating activities right before bed.
- To relieve tension, practice relaxation techniques like deep breathing or meditation.
- Avoid drinking and eating large meals right before bed.
- If you're having trouble sleeping, think about getting advice and an assessment from a medical professional or sleep specialist. The

ability to sleep is essential for good health, and treating sleep-related issues can have a significant effect on hormone balance and general wellbeing.

Chapter 4: Techniques for Hormone Balancing

A. Herbal supplements and natural remedies

A lot of people use herbal supplements and natural therapies to support many aspects of their health, including hormone balance. It's crucial to remember that even while some herbal supplements and natural cures could be beneficial, you should use them sparingly and speak with a doctor before introducing them into your regimen.

The following herbal medicines and home cures are occasionally used to promote hormonal health:

1. Black cohosh: Women frequently take this herb to reduce menopausal symptoms including mood swings and hot flashes.

2. Vitex agnus-castus, or chasteberry, is said to help control the menstrual cycle and lessen premenstrual syndrome symptoms (PMS).

3. Soy Isoflavones: These plant-based phytoestrogens may alleviate menopausal symptoms and promote women's estrogen balance.

4. Maca Root: Helps balance hormones, increase libido, and support energy levels.

5. Ashwagandha: An adaptogen that could boost thyroid function and aid in stress management.

6. Dong Quai: Traditionally used in Chinese medicine to promote hormonal balance and ease menstrual discomfort.

7. Gamma-linolenic acid (GLA) is found in evening primrose oil, which is used for its possible ability to help with PMS symptoms.

8. Saw palmetto: Supposed to help men's prostate health and may affect the sex hormone balance.

9. Diosgenin, which can occasionally be utilized to make synthetic hormones, is present in wild yam. It has long been used to relieve menopausal symptoms and discomfort associated with the menstrual cycle.

10. Some women use red clover, which contains phytoestrogens, to ease the symptoms of menopause.

11. Rhodiola rosea: An adaptogenic herb that promotes general wellbeing and may assist the body in adjusting to stress.

12. Licorice Root: May support cortisol balance and adrenal health.

13. Ginseng: Known as an adaptogen, ginseng may promote general health and assist the body in adjusting to stress.

14. Fenugreek: Supposed to aid in hormonal balance and blood sugar regulation.

15. Cinnamon: May aid in controlling insulin sensitivity and blood sugar levels.

16. Curcumin, an anti-inflammatory compound found in turmeric, may benefit general health.

17. Some women use sage to relieve menopausal symptoms, especially hot flashes.

18. Nettle Root: May support hormonal balance and men's prostate health.

19. Nutrients found in stinging nettle may help maintain hormonal balance and general wellness.

20. Milk Thistle: May promote liver health, which may have an indirect effect on the metabolism of hormones.

It's important to use caution when utilizing herbal supplements and natural therapies, and to speak with a healthcare professional beforehand if you take medication or have underlying medical concerns. These treatments may have unforeseen negative effects or interfere with medication. Furthermore, individual differences exist in the efficacy of herbal supplements, and further studies are frequently required to confirm their safety and usefulness.

Keep in mind that the foundation of hormonal health is a balanced diet, consistent exercise, enough sleep, and stress management. Herbs and natural therapies can be a great addition to a healthy lifestyle, but they shouldn't be the only thing you use to treat hormonal imbalances or other health issues.

B.	Treatment	with	Hormone Replacement (HRT)

A medical procedure known as hormone replacement therapy (HRT) entails adding new hormones to the body in order to correct hormonal imbalances or treat symptoms brought on by these changes. It is most frequently used to treat menopausal symptoms in women, but it can be applied in a variety of other contexts as well. This is a summary of HRT:

1. Hormone Replacement Therapy for Menopause:

Menopausal hormone replacement therapy (HRT) is used to treat menopausal symptoms such as hot flashes, vaginal dryness, and mood swings. In order to lower the risk of uterine cancer, it usually entails estrogen replacement and, if a woman still retains her uterus, may also include progestin, a synthetic form of progesterone. There are various kinds, such as:

- Estrogen-only therapy: Usually recommended for female patients who have undergone hysterectomy (uterine removal).
- Combining progestin and estrogen therapy: Suggested for females who still have an intact uterus.

2. Men's Hormone Replacement:

- Men with low testosterone levels (hypogonadism) can treat symptoms like muscle loss, exhaustion, and decreased libido with testosterone replacement medication. It is applied as patches, gels, or injections.

3. Thyroid Hormone Substitute:

- Thyroid conditions like hypothyroidism (underactive thyroid) and hyperthyroidism (overactive thyroid) are treated with this therapy. To reestablish equilibrium, doctors administer synthetic thyroid hormones.

4. Adrenal Hormone Substitute:

- Glucocorticoid and mineralocorticoid replacement therapy are administered to treat patients with Addison's disease, or adrenal insufficiency, in order to replenish the hormones that the adrenal glands are unable to generate.

5. Growth Hormone Substitute:

- When a person has a growth hormone shortage, usually in children but occasionally in adults, growth hormone replacement treatment is done. It promotes development and growth.

6. Hormone Substitution for Gender Shift:

- Those undergoing gender transition can acquire secondary sexual traits that are compatible with their gender identity with the use of hormone replacement treatment. Hormones including estrogen and testosterone are administered in this process.

7. Hormone therapy for osteoporosis:

- Postmenopausal women may utilize estrogen or estrogen-progestin treatment to prevent or treat osteoporosis. It sustains the density of the bones.

It's crucial to remember that HRT can have risks as well as advantages, and that a person's age, health, and particular hormone imbalance will all determine whether or not it is safe to use. An increased risk of certain medical disorders, such as blood clots, stroke, and breast cancer, is one of the risks linked to hormone replacement therapy.

Consequently, choices on hormone replacement therapy (HRT) must be made following a comprehensive assessment by a medical professional, who will also take into account the patient's particular situation and risk factors.

To maximize benefits and minimize hazards, a healthcare professional should prescribe, monitor, and modify hormone replacement therapy (HRT). It is usually necessary to schedule follow-up sessions on a regular basis in order to monitor the patient's reaction to therapy and identify any possible side effects. When thinking about HRT, it's critical to have honest and knowledgeable conversations with your healthcare physician.

C.   Alternative   Medicine   (Yoga, Acupuncture, etc.)

Acupuncture, yoga, and other complementary therapies are examples of alternative therapies that are frequently used to improve hormonal balance and, in certain situations, to enhance general well-being. These therapies can be combined with traditional medical treatments or used as part of a holistic approach to health.

An outline of some well-liked complementary therapies and how they could affect hormonal health is provided below:

1. Chinese medicine

- The traditional Chinese medical procedure known as acupuncture involves inserting tiny needles into predetermined bodily locations. It is thought to assist in controlling the body's Qi, or energy flow. Acupuncture may help regulate hormones, lowering cortisol and increasing calm, according to some research. It's frequently used to treat a range of medical conditions, such as stress, fertility, and menopausal symptoms.

2. Posha:

Yoga promotes flexibility, strength, and relaxation by combining physical postures, breathing techniques, and meditation. It has the potential to lower cortisol and stress levels. Backbends and inversions are two examples of yoga positions that may stimulate the endocrine system and support hormonal balance. Yoga is frequently used to treat hormone imbalance symptoms, maintain thyroid function, and reduce stress.

3. Mindfulness & Meditation:

- Deep relaxation methods and focused concentration are key components of mindfulness and meditation practices. These techniques can support hormonal balance, lower cortisol levels, and lessen stress. Programs for mindfulness-based stress reduction (MBSR) are useful in treating hormone imbalances brought on by stress.

4. Chi Gong:

- Tai Chi is a slow-moving, peaceful Chinese martial art that combines meditation, awareness, and fluid motions. It can lessen stress and enhance general wellbeing. Although further research is required, Tai Chi has been proposed as a possible method to help balance hormones.

5. In Ayurveda:

- The goal of India's ancient Ayurvedic medical system is to balance the body's energies and preserve general health. In order to support hormonal balance, it comprises dietary and lifestyle suggestions as well as the use of vitamins and herbs. Herbs used in Ayurveda medicine, such as Shatavari and ashwagandha, are used to treat hormonal problems, such as menopause symptoms and stress.

6. Herbal Remedies:

- Herbal therapies can be utilized to improve hormonal balance. Examples of these include phytoestrogen-rich plants (like black cohosh and red clover), adaptogenic herbs (such ashwagandha and Rhodiola), and traditional herbal formulae. Herbal medicines should always be used under the guidance of a trained herbalist or healthcare professional, especially when used in conjunction with other therapies.

7. Essential oils:

- Aromatherapy uses essential oils to promote relaxation and elevate mood. Certain essential oils, such as clary sage and lavender, are thought to offer potential advantages in the treatment of hormone imbalances and stress. They can be diluted and applied topically, or they can be utilized in diffusers.

It's crucial to remember that each person may respond differently to these alternative therapies, so they shouldn't be used in place of traditional medical care when it's appropriate. Before beginning any new treatment or supplement, always get medical advice, especially if you have underlying medical conditions or are taking medication.

A comprehensive strategy for regulating hormonal balance and general well-being can be obtained through an integrated approach to health, which blends complementary and alternative therapies with traditional medicine.

Chapter 5: Hormonal Balance Dietary Solutions

Nutrient-Rich Foods

Eating foods high in nutrients is crucial to preserving hormonal balance and general wellness. The body receives vital vitamins, minerals, antioxidants, and other chemicals from these foods to support a range of physiological processes, including hormone regulation. The following is a list of foods high in nutrients that you ought to think about including in your diet:

1. Berries:

- Berries: High in fiber, vitamins, and antioxidants, including blueberries, strawberries, and raspberries.

- Citrus fruits (grapefruits, oranges, and lemons): Rich in fiber and vitamin C.

- Avocado: Rich in several vitamins and good fats.

- Apples: Rich in antioxidants, vitamins, and fiber.

2. Vegetables

- Leafy greens: A great source of antioxidants, vitamins, and minerals are spinach, kale, and Swiss chard.

- Cruciferous vegetables: Brussels sprouts, cauliflower, and broccoli: include substances that help maintain hormone balance.
Carrots: High in fiber and beta-carotene.

- Sweet potatoes: Rich in complex carbs, fiber, and vitamins.

3. Complete Grains:

- Oats: Rich in complex carbs and fiber.

-Quinoa: Packed full of vitamins and minerals, it's a complete protein source.
- Brown rice: Provides vital minerals and fiber.

- Whole wheat pasta and bread: Excellent providers of B vitamins and fiber.

4. Reduced Proteins:

- Salmon: high-quality protein and omega-3 fatty acid-rich seafood.

- Skinless poultry, such as turkey and chicken, are lean protein sources.

- Tofu and tempeh: Plant-based sources of critical amino acids in protein.

- Legumes: Rich in protein and fiber, such as beans and lentils.

5. Seeds and Nuts:

- Almonds, walnuts, and flaxseeds: Offer vital nutrients, fiber, and good fats.

- Chia seeds: High in fiber and omega-3 fatty acids.

- Sunflower seeds: Packed in minerals and vitamin E.

6. Dairy and its Substitutes:

- Greek yogurt: Packed with probiotics and protein.

- Soy or almond milk that has been fortified: Excellent providers of calcium and vitamin D.

- Low-fat cheese: Provides protein and calcium.

7. Eggs:

- Eggs offer a variety of vitamins and minerals and are a full protein source.

8. Trim Meats:

- Lean beef and pork slices are excellent providers of iron, protein, and other necessary elements.

9. seafood

- In addition to salmon, seafood such as mussels and shrimp provide vital minerals and lean protein.

10. Grains:

- Plant-based sources of fiber and protein include beans, lentils, and chickpeas.

11. Spices and Herbs:

- Turmeric: This spice possesses an anti-inflammatory compound called curcumin.

- Cinnamon: This spice may aid in blood sugar regulation.

12. Verdant Tea

Antioxidants and other chemicals that may improve general health are abundant in green tea.

13. Alternatives to Dairy:

- Almond milk, soy milk, and other dairy substitutes that have been enhanced with calcium and vitamin D.

14. Olive Oil

- Extra virgin olive oil is a good source of antioxidants and monounsaturated fats.

15. Garlic

- Allicin, a substance found in garlic, may be beneficial to health.

These nutrient-rich foods can be included in a well-balanced diet to give your body the vital nutrients it needs to support general health, maintain hormonal balance, and lower the risk of hormonal imbalances and related health problems.

It's important to remember to stay hydrated during the day by drinking lots of water, as this is also essential for general health.

A.   Hormone-Related   Dietary Strategies

Eating a hormone-supportive diet entails selecting foods that promote overall health and hormonal balance. While dietary requirements can differ from person to person, there are several eating habits and concepts that are linked to hormonal health. Consider the following hormone-supportive diets:

1. Balanced Diet:

- Nutrient-dense foods from all dietary groups, such as fruits, vegetables, whole grains, lean meats, and healthy fats, are included in a balanced diet. This method aids in supplying vital nutrients for maintaining hormonal equilibrium.

2. Mediterranean Diet:

- Fruits, vegetables, whole grains, fish, nuts, and olive oil are abundant in the Mediterranean diet. It may promote hormonal health and is linked to decreased incidence of heart disease.

3.. Low-Glycemic Diet:

- Foods with little effect on blood sugar levels are the main emphasis of a low-glycemic diet. Lean proteins, non-starchy veggies, legumes, and whole grains are all included. This strategy can assist in controlling cortisol and insulin levels.

4. Anti-Inflammatory Diet:

- Foods high in omega-3 fatty acids, fruits, vegetables, nuts, and spices like turmeric are highlights of an anti-inflammatory diet. Reducing inflammation can be helpful because it can throw off the hormonal balance.

5. Plant-Based Diet

- The main components of a plant-based diet are whole grains, legumes, fruits, and vegetables. Hormone balance is one aspect of general health that it can support.

6. Whole Foods Diet:

- The goal of this strategy is to prioritize whole, unprocessed foods while reducing the amount of processed and refined meals. It guarantees the consumption of vital nutrients and helps maintain hormonal equilibrium.

7. High-Fiber Diet

- Fiber-rich foods including fruits, vegetables, whole grains, and legumes can support healthy digestion and help control blood sugar levels, which can have an indirect impact on hormonal balance.

8. DASH Diet:

- The Dietary Approaches to Stop Hypertension (DASH) diet places a strong emphasis on consuming more fruits, vegetables, whole grains, lean meats, low-fat dairy, and lowering sodium intake. It can help control hormones linked to blood pressure and promote general health.

9. Hormone-Specific Diets:

- In certain situations, eating regimens tailored to address specific hormonal abnormalities may be advised. For example, a low-iodine diet or a low-sugar diet may be recommended for people with thyroid problems or insulin resistance, respectively.

10. Intermittent Fasting:

When done correctly, some people discover that intermittent fasting can help control insulin levels and support hormonal balance. It entails eating and fasting cycles.

11. Mindful Eating:

- Mindful eating is a technique that emphasizes observing signals of hunger and fullness and indulging in food without interruption. In addition to promoting hormonal balance that affects appetite regulation, this may assist avoid overindulging.

It's crucial to remember that every person has different nutritional requirements and tastes, so the ideal eating schedule for you will rely on your unique health objectives and hormone issues. Speak with a medical professional or qualified dietitian to develop a customized nutrition plan that takes into account your particular requirements. In addition, any food strategy to enhance general hormonal balance should be complemented by lifestyle factors like exercise, stress reduction, and sleep.

Chapter 6: Exercise and Hormonal Balance

A. Significance of Regular Physical Activities

Engaging in regular physical activity is crucial for maintaining general health and wellbeing. It is essential for supporting mental, emotional, and physical well-being and is intimately related to hormone control in the body. Here are some main arguments supporting the significance of routine physical activity:

1. Hormone Equilibrium:

- By encouraging the appropriate release of insulin, cortisol, thyroid hormones, and sex hormones including estrogen and testosterone, exercise aids in hormone regulation. Hormonal imbalances can be prevented with regular exercise.

2. Maintaining Weight:

- By raising metabolic rate and burning calories, physical activity helps with weight control. Hormonal equilibrium depends on maintaining a healthy weight because extra body fat can throw hormone levels out of balance.

3. Heart-Related Health:

Frequent exercise lowers the risk of heart disease and associated hormone imbalances by strengthening the heart and circulation system.

4. Blood Sugar Management:

- Exercise improves the body's sensitivity to insulin, which aids with blood sugar regulation. For those who have diabetes or insulin resistance, this is extremely crucial.

5. Bone Wellness:

- Weight-bearing activities that preserve bone density and lower the chance of hormone abnormalities associated with osteoporosis include walking and strength training.

6. Hormones and Strength of Muscle:

- Strength training contributes to the growth and maintenance of muscle mass, which, particularly as people age, can positively impact hormone balance.

7. Mental Wellness:

- Engaging in physical activity causes the production of endorphins, which elevate mood and lessen depressive and anxious symptoms. Exercise affects hormones such as dopamine and serotonin.

8. Stress Reduction:

Frequent exercise aids in stress management and reduction for the body. It can help with the hormonal abnormalities brought on by prolonged stress and lower cortisol levels.

9. Conditions Connected to Hormones:

- Hormone-related diseases like polycystic ovarian syndrome (PCOS), menopausal symptoms, and hormone-related malignancies can all be prevented and managed with exercise.

10. Sleep Standard:

- Exercise improves sleep patterns by indirectly affecting the balance of hormones, which includes the regulation of melatonin and cortisol.

11. Immune System:

Frequent, moderate-intensity exercise helps strengthen the body's defenses against infections by boosting the immune system's performance.

12. Mental Process:

- Brain-derived neurotrophic factor (BDNF), a protein that resembles a hormone and supports brain health, is released when physical exercise occurs. This enhances cognitive function, memory, and brain health.

13. Durability:

- A longer lifespan and better aging are linked to exercise. It may lessen the likelihood of hormonal abnormalities brought on by aging.

14. Emotional Health:

Frequent exercise promotes mental toughness, self-worth, and a sense of accomplishment, all of which are beneficial for hormone balance and emotional health.

15. Social Communication:

- Group exercise, sports, and fitness courses offer chances for social support and interaction, which can have a positive effect on mental and emotional health.

Selecting physical activities that you enjoy and can stick with over time is key. Exercises ranging from aerobic to strength training to flexibility can offer a comprehensive approach to hormone balance and general wellness. Before beginning a new fitness regimen, always get medical advice, especially if you have any underlying health issues or concerns.

B. Types of Exercises for Hormone Regulation

Exercises of all kinds can have a favorable impact on how the body regulates hormones. The type of exercise you choose should be determined by your own tastes, level of fitness, and specific health objectives. The following activities can help maintain hormonal balance:

1.   Cardiovascular   or   Aerobic Workouts:

- Running: This high-impact aerobic activity has a good effect on hormone control while also lowering stress and enhancing cardiovascular health.

- Cycling: Cycling is a fantastic way to increase endurance and control hormones, whether you do it outside or on a stationary cycle.

- Swimming: This low-impact activity helps lower stress and increase cardiovascular fitness.

- Dancing: Dancing is an enjoyable and sociable method to raise your heart rate, improve your mood, and maintain hormonal equilibrium.

- Brisk Walking: This easy-to-learn but efficient workout is good for all fitness levels and can aid with stress relief and weight management.

2. Strength Exercise:

- Weight Lifting: Building and maintaining muscle mass through strength training, which includes weight lifting and resistance exercises, helps hormonal balance.

- Bodyweight Exercises: By using your own body weight as resistance, exercises like push-ups, squats, and planks can help you strengthen your bones and gain muscle.

- Yoga: Although mostly a flexibility practice, some yoga poses and styles can help support hormonal balance by including strength training components.

3. HIIT, or high-intensity interval training:

HIIT alternates brief intervals of high-intensity training with rest intervals. By boosting the synthesis of growth hormone, enhancing insulin sensitivity, and encouraging weight control, it can aid in hormone regulation.

4. Exercises for Flexibility and Balance:

- Yoga: Beyond its strength training components, yoga promotes balance and flexibility, which can aid in stress reduction and general wellbeing.

- Pilates: Pilates offers a comprehensive approach to hormonal health by emphasizing balance, flexibility, and strength in the core.

5. Body-Mind Exercises:

- Tai Chi: This kind of meditation and gentle, flowing movements is combined with deep breathing. It can enhance hormone regulation, balance, and lessen stress.

- Qigong: Like Tai Chi, Qigong promotes relaxation and stress reduction by combining breathing exercises, meditation, and gentle movements.

6. Intermittent Exercise and Fasting:

- The metabolic and hormonal advantages of both intermittent fasting and exercise can be increased. Exercise after a fast can enhance insulin sensitivity and support hormone balance.

7. Relaxation techniques

Deep breathing techniques, progressive muscle relaxation, and mindfulness meditation are a few practices that can assist with stress management, cortisol reduction, and hormone balance.

Consistency is the key to efficient exercise for hormone management. The World Health Organization recommends doing at least 150 minutes of moderate-intensity aerobic activity, 75 minutes of vigorous-intensity aerobic exercise, or a combination of both, each week. Maintaining muscle mass can also be aided by doing strength training activities at least twice a week.

Before beginning a new workout regimen, it is imperative that you speak with a healthcare provider or fitness expert, particularly if you have any underlying medical concerns. To maintain hormonal balance through physical activity, the best option may be to create a customized exercise plan that fits your goals and your degree of fitness.

Chapter 7: Stress Management Techniques

A. Meditation and Mindfulness

Self-awareness, relaxation techniques, and focused attention are all part of mindfulness and meditation practices. They can make a significant difference in lowering stress, enhancing emotional health, and fostering hormonal balance. An outline of the advantages of mindfulness and meditation for hormone regulation is provided below:

1. Being mindful:

Being totally present in the moment, without distraction or judgment, is the practice of mindfulness. It entails being aware of your ideas, emotions, physical sensations, and external circumstances.

Advantages for Hormone Balance:

- Stress Reduction: By assisting people in better controlling how they respond to stimuli, mindfulness can help people feel less stressed. The body's main stress hormone, cortisol, decreases in response to reduced stress levels.

- Emotional management: Mindfulness has the potential to lessen mood disorders and enhance emotional management. Mood disorders and other hormone-related illnesses may benefit from this.

- Insulin Sensitivity: Research indicates that mindfulness exercises may enhance insulin sensitivity, a crucial factor in hormone balance and blood sugar control.

- Better Sleep: Practicing mindfulness can help you unwind and get a better night's sleep, which can contribute to better hormone control, including higher levels of cortisol and melatonin.

2. Reflection:

- Meditation is a mental practice that promotes focus and profound relaxation. There are many different kinds of meditation, such as transcendental, loving-kindness, and mindfulness meditation.

Advantages for Hormone Balance:

- Stress Reduction: One effective method for controlling stress and reducing cortisol levels is meditation. Decreased stress can benefit general wellbeing and hormone balance.

- Brain Health: Studies have shown a connection between enhanced brain health and specific meditation techniques. This includes the production of brain-derived neurotrophic factor (BDNF), which promotes emotional stability and cognitive performance.

- Sleep Improvement: Meditation helps promote better hormonal balance, especially melatonin levels, by relaxing the body and mind. This makes it easier to go asleep and stay asleep.

- Blood Pressure Regulation: Mindfulness and other meditation techniques can lower blood pressure, which is important for hormone balance and cardiovascular health.

How to Combine Meditation and Mindfulness:

- Locate a Calm Area: Pick a peaceful, distraction-free area where you can sit or lie down.

- Set Aside Time: Designate a particular period of time for your meditation or mindfulness exercises. Every day, even a little while can have advantages.

- Start with Breath Awareness: Pay attention to your breath at first. As you inhale and exhale, become aware of how your breath feels.

- Mindful Body Scan: This technique helps you relax and release tension by gradually focusing your attention on various body areas.

- Guided Meditations: To help you get started and keep up your practice, you can use guided meditation apps, movies, or recordings.

- Have patience: Meditation and mindfulness are practices that take time to master. If your thoughts stray, don't give up; just softly refocus on the area you have selected.

- Consistency: To get the benefits, practice consistently. Create a schedule that suits your needs.

To maintain hormonal balance, mindfulness and meditation can be utilized alone or in conjunction with other stress-reduction strategies like consistent exercise. These techniques are useful for enhancing general wellbeing and minimizing the negative effects of stress on hormone control.

A. Meditation Activities

Stress reduction, hormone balance, and physical and mental relaxation are all supported by relaxation activities. Taking part in these activities can improve general wellbeing. You can try these relaxation techniques:

1. Deep Inhalation:

Comfortably lie down or sit.
- Breathe slowly and deeply via your nose, raising your abdomen in the process.

- Gently exhale through your mouth to ensure that your lungs are entirely empty.

- Keep breathing deeply while paying attention to it and releasing tension with each exhale.

2. Progressive Relaxation of Muscles:

- Begin with your toes and work your way up, or start at the top and work your way down.

- For a few seconds, tense and then release each muscle group, allowing the tension to dissolve.

- As you move through your body, notice how tension and relaxation differ from one another.

3. Suggested Imagery:

Shut your eyes and visualize a serene, contemplative location, like a woodland, beach, or meadow.

- Precisely visualize the scenario using all of your senses, including the sounds, scents, and sensations.

- Allow your body and mind to unwind as you immerse yourself in this mental oasis.

4. Autonomous Instruction:

- Recite a few words or affirmations aloud while in a comfortable position. Examples include "My right arm is heavy and warm" and "I am calm and at peace."

- Pay attention to the feelings evoked by these claims and use them to help you relax.

5. Concise Coloring:

- Use coloring books that are intended to be relaxing.

- Let your thoughts relax and focus on the process of coloring, taking note of the hues, forms, and patterns.

6. Nidra Yoga:

- A guided meditation and relaxation technique in which you gradually relax various body areas while keeping your awareness of your breath and sensations.

7. Qigong or Tai Chi:

- To encourage balance and relaxation, these mind-body techniques combine deep breathing with soft, flowing motions.

8. Writing a Journal:

- Expressing your ideas and feelings via writing can be a therapeutic method to lower stress and enhance mental health.

9. Hot Bath:

- To relax and release stress, soak in a warm bath using Epsom salts or fragrant oils.

10. Musical Therapy:

- To relax and lower stress, listen to peaceful instrumental music or the sounds of nature.

11. Essential oils:

- To create a relaxing ambiance, use essential oils like lavender or chamomile in a diffuser or as part of a relaxation routine.

12. Illustration:

- Visualize yourself in a calm and serene environment. Imagine the specifics, then let the calmness envelope you.

13. Guided Relaxation Apps and Recordings:

- To help you relax, a lot of apps and internet resources include guided breathing techniques and meditation sessions.

14. Nature Stroll:

- Take time to enjoy the outdoors, be it a park, forest, or beach. Establishing a connection with the natural world can be incredibly soothing.

It's critical to identify the relaxation techniques that are most effective for you and incorporate them into your daily practice. Reducing stress's negative effects on hormone control, enhancing mental stability, and promoting general health are all possible with relaxation techniques.

D. Reducing Stress in Everyday Life

Reducing stress in daily life is essential for preserving hormonal balance, as well as for mental and physical health. Prolonged stress can negatively affect your hormones and general well-being. The following are some practical methods to lessen stress in day-to-day living:

1. Meditation & Mindfulness:

- Regularly engage in mindfulness and meditation techniques to maintain mental clarity and present-moment awareness. Stress can be significantly reduced by engaging in guided meditation or deep breathing exercises for even a short while.

2. Engaging in Exercise:

- Get regular exercise, whether it be yoga, jogging, walking, or any other physical activity you enjoy. Endorphins are naturally occurring hormones that are released during exercise.

3. Optimal Diet:

Eat a diet high in nutrient-dense, well-balanced meals. A healthy diet aids in hormone balance and improves your body's ability to handle stress.

4. Rest:

Make sleep a priority by planning a regular sleep schedule and developing a calming nighttime routine. Hormone balance and stress control depend on getting enough sleep.

5. Time Handling:

- Set priorities for your duties and organize your chores. Feelings of overwhelm can be lessened with good time management.

6. Social Assistance:

- Maintain social and emotional ties with friends and family to foster interaction. Stress can be reduced by talking to loved ones about your feelings.

7. Unwinding Methods:

- Include relaxation techniques in your regimen, like progressive muscle relaxation, deep breathing, and warm baths.

8. Limit alcohol and caffeine:

Limit alcohol and caffeine intake as these substances can aggravate stress and interfere with sleep cycles.

9. Cut Down on Screen Time:

- Take pauses from social media and electronics to lessen the risk of stress and information overload.

10. Develop Your Gratitude:

- Express your gratitude for items on a regular basis. A thankfulness notebook is a great resource for developing optimism.

11. Establish Limits:

- Acquire the ability to decline new obligations when you're feeling overburdened. One of the most crucial aspects of stress management is setting boundaries.

12. Organize and Declutter:

- An orderly and clean space helps lessen tension and feelings of disarray.

13. Seek Expert Assistance:

Please don't hesitate to get assistance from a therapist, counselor, or mental health professional if stress is having a substantial negative influence on your life.

14. Conscious Eating:

- Engage in mindful eating by focusing solely on your meals while avoiding outside distractions. It can make eating more enjoyable for you and lessen stress-related overeating.

15. Laughing

- Take part in humorous activities, such as viewing a humorous film, reading a humorous book, or hanging out with happy people.

16. Outdoors and Fresh Air:

- Take a walk outside, spend time in nature, or just breathe in some fresh air. Being in tune with nature may be very calming.

17. Interests and Hobbies:

- Set aside time for passion-driven pursuits and hobbies. Taking part in things you enjoy might be a healthy way to decompress.

18. Develop Your Resilience:

- Reframe stress to help you become more resilient. Strive to view obstacles as chances for development and education.

19. Gratitude-based statements:

- Use constructive self-talk to combat negative self-talk and cultivate an optimistic outlook.

20. Professional Support:

- Seek assistance from a mental health expert as soon as possible if your stress is taking a toll on your life. They can offer direction and support.

Though everyone feels stress, how you handle it has a big influence on your overall health. To maintain hormonal balance and general health, it's critical to identify the stress-reduction techniques that are most effective for you and incorporate them into your daily routine.

Chapter 8: Hormonal Health and Sleep

A. The Importance of Good Sleep

Getting a good night's sleep is crucial for general health and wellbeing. It is essential for everyday functioning, physical and mental health, and hormone regulation. This is why getting enough sleep is so important:

1. Hormonal Equilibrium:

- Hormone control and sleep are closely related. Your sleep patterns affect many hormones, including growth hormone, insulin, cortisol, and leptin. These hormone cycles can be upset by getting poor-quality sleep, which may result in imbalances.

2. The role of the immune system

- A healthy immune system depends on getting enough sleep. The body produces cytokine proteins that support the immune response when it gets enough sleep. Your immune system might be weakened by sleep deprivation, leaving you more vulnerable to sickness.

3. Mental Processes:

- Cognitive processes like memory, focus, creativity, and problem-solving depend on getting enough sleep. It enables the brain to digest information from the day and combine memories.

4. Welfare of the Emotions:

- Getting enough sleep is essential for controlling emotions. It lessens the likelihood of mood disorders including anxiety and sadness and supports the maintenance of a cheerful attitude.

5. Health of the Body:

- Blood sugar regulation, weight control, and cardiovascular health are among the physical health aspects that are linked to sleep. Long-term sleep deprivation has been associated with a higher risk of diabetes, obesity, and heart disease.

6. Restoration and Regrowth:

- The body heals, grows, and regenerates itself when you are in deep sleep. The body heals its bones, muscles, and tissues while we sleep.

7. Production of Hormones:

- Getting enough sleep helps the body produce growth hormone, which is essential for maintaining and repairing physical growth. Furthermore, sleep influences hunger and satiety cues by regulating hormones linked to appetite.

8. Stress Reduction:

- Sleep is essential for managing stress. Cortisol levels, which can rise with sleep loss, can be lowered and the body's stress response can be regulated with adequate rest.

9. Vitality & Energy:

- Getting a good night's sleep is crucial to waking up refreshed and focused. It promotes both mental and physical health, making you more concentrated and productive.

10. Pain Control:

- Sleep can improve the body's capacity to tolerate discomfort and lessen the sense of pain. It's crucial for people who are managing chronic pain disorders in particular.

11. Conditions Connected to Hormones:

- Adequate sleep is beneficial for hormonal illnesses like polycystic ovarian syndrome (PCOS), thyroid abnormalities, and adrenal problems because it balances and controls hormone production.

12. Lifespan:

- A longer and healthier life expectancy is linked to a regular sleep schedule of high quality.

Consider implementing good sleep hygiene habits to encourage restful sleep, such as sticking to a regular sleep schedule, setting up a cozy sleeping space, minimizing screen time before bed, and consuming moderate amounts of alcohol and caffeine. Seek advice and examination from a healthcare provider or sleep specialist if you experience recurring sleep issues. The foundation of good health is getting enough sleep, which is crucial for preserving hormonal balance, mental clarity, and emotional stability.

B. Sleep Hygiene Tips

A collection of behaviors and habits that support restful sleep is referred to as sleep hygiene. You may sleep longer, go to sleep earlier, and wake up feeling more rested by practicing better sleep hygiene. Here are some suggestions for good sleep hygiene:

1. Keep a Regular Sleep Schedule:

- Set a regular wake-up and bedtime every day, including on the weekends. Your body's internal clock can be regulated with consistency.

2. Establish a Calm Bedtime Schedule:

- Create a relaxing routine before bed. This could involve engaging in relaxing activities like reading, having a warm bath, or doing yoga.

3. Create a Comfortable Sleep Environment

Make sure you have a sleeping-friendly bedroom. This calls for a cold environment with comfy pillows and mattresses, as well as little light and noise. If needed, think about using a sleep mask or blackout curtains.

4. Minimize Screen Time:

- The blue light that computers, tablets, and cell phones emit can disrupt your sleep-wake cycle. At least one hour before going to bed, avoid using screens.

5. Pay Attention to What You Consume:

- Steer clear of large or spicy foods right before bed since they may make you uncomfortable. Restrict your intake of alcohol and caffeine, especially in the hours before bed.

6. Exercise Frequently:

Frequent exercise can enhance the quality of your sleep, but avoid intense exercise right before bed because it may be stimulating.

7. Stress Management:

- Anxiety and stress might make it hard to fall asleep. To relax, use stress-reduction methods like progressive muscle relaxation, deep breathing, or meditation.

8. Restrict Naps:

- If you must take a nap during the day, limit it to 20 to 30 minutes, and stay away from naps in the late afternoon as these can disrupt your sleep at night.

9. Minimize Drinking Before Sleep:

Reduce the amount of fluids you drink, especially right before bed, to lessen the chance that you'll wake up in the middle of the night to use the restroom.

10. Make Time in Your Bed for Sleep and Closeness:

- Refrain from doing tasks like working or watching TV in bed. Your body will become more accustomed to relaxing when you enter your bed if you associate it with sleep.

11. Control Your Daylight Exposure:

- During the day, exposure to natural light aids in sleep-wake cycle regulation. Spend time outside, preferably early in the day, to improve your circadian cycle.

12. Continue to Move Throughout the Day:

Frequent exercise can enhance the quality of your sleep, but avoid intense exercise right before bed because it may be stimulating.

13. Speak with a Medical Expert:

- If, after attempting these suggestions, you still have trouble falling asleep or if you have a sleep condition, see a doctor or sleep specialist for a comprehensive assessment and advice.

Remember that enhancing sleep hygiene frequently necessitates making mistakes. It's critical to identify the routines and habits that are most effective for you. You may greatly improve your sleep and general well-being by making excellent sleep a priority and putting these suggestions into practice.

Chapter 9: Hormonal Disproportion in Various Life Stages

Both men and women can be affected by hormonal abnormalities at different phases of life. Numerous factors, such as age, health conditions, genetics, and lifestyle choices, might contribute to these imbalances. An outline of hormone imbalances at various phases of life is provided below:

1. Puberty: During this phase of life, teenagers undergo notable hormonal changes, such as elevated levels of sex hormones (testosterone and estrogen). Hormonal changes cause emotional and physical changes, including mood

swings and the emergence of secondary sexual traits.

2. Reproductive Years: - Women: Endometriosis, irregular menstrual periods, and polycystic ovarian syndrome (PCOS) can all be brought on by hormonal abnormalities at this time. During this phase, menopause and pregnancy are also important hormonal turning points.

- males: During their reproductive years, males may have hormonal imbalances, such as low testosterone, which can result in symptoms like exhaustion and decreased libido.

3. Postpartum and Pregnancy: - Significant hormonal changes occur during pregnancy, especially increases

in progesterone and estrogen, which promote fetal development. Many women undergo postpartum hormone changes after giving birth, which may be a factor in mood disorders including postpartum depression.

4. Andropause and Menopause: Women usually experience the menopause, or the end of their menstrual cycle, in their late 40s or early 50s. It causes estrogen and progesterone levels to drop, which can cause a variety of symptoms like mood swings, hot flashes, and a decrease of bone density.

Andropause, sometimes known as "male menopause," is the progressive reduction in testosterone levels that occurs in older men. It may result in symptoms such as decreased muscular mass, low energy, and sexual dysfunction.

5. Aging: Hormonal changes are linked to aging in both men and women. When women get closer to menopause, their levels of estrogen drop, causing a variety of symptoms. As men age, their levels of testosterone likewise gradually decline, which can have an effect on their sexual function, bone density, and muscle mass.

6. Adrenal insufficiency: Disorders such as Addison's disease can result in an insufficiency of the adrenal glands, which can cause imbalances in the hormones cortisol and aldosterone that are produced by the glands. This may lead to symptoms such as

electrolyte imbalances, low blood pressure, and weariness.

7. Thyroid diseases: - Men and women are both susceptible to thyroid diseases, which include hyperthyroidism and hypothyroidism, which can arise at any age. These disorders cause thyroid hormone abnormalities, which can cause symptoms like mood swings, exhaustion, and weight fluctuations.

8. Hormonal Cancers: - A number of cancers, including those of the breast, prostate, and ovary, are caused by hormones. Often, hormone imbalance management or disruption techniques are part of the treatment for these tumors.

9. Lifestyle and Environmental variables: - Lifestyle variables, including poor diet, inactivity, long-term stress, and exposure to pollutants in the environment, can also have an impact on hormonal imbalances.

Depending on the exact disease and time of life, treating hormonal imbalances may entail lifestyle modifications, medicines, hormone replacement treatment, or surgical procedures. If you believe you may have a hormonal imbalance or are experiencing symptoms associated with swings in your hormone levels, it is crucial that you seek the advice and comprehensive evaluation of a healthcare professional.

Chapter 10: Hormonal Balance and Women's Health

A. Effects on Pregnancy and Fertility

In both men and women, hormonal abnormalities can have a major effect on fertility and pregnancy. These imbalances may affect an individual's overall reproductive health as well as the procedures required for conception and a healthy pregnancy. Hormonal imbalances can impact pregnancy and fertility in the following ways:

Effect on Pregnancy and Fertility:

1. irregular Menstrual Cycles: Irregular menstrual cycles can be caused by hormonal imbalances, such as those caused by thyroid conditions or polycystic ovarian syndrome (PCOS), which can make it challenging to anticipate ovulation and become pregnant.

2. Anovulation: A number of hormonal disorders can interfere with the normal release of eggs during ovulation. Anovulation, or the lack of ovulation, is a frequent problem that can result in infertility in women who have hormonal imbalances.

3. Luteal Phase Defect: This is a condition in which the second half of the menstrual cycle is shortened due to an imbalance in hormones. A fertilized

egg may have difficulty implanting in the uterus as a result of this abnormality.

4. Uterine Problems: Imbalances in hormones can disrupt the uterine lining, which can affect the uterus's capacity to support a pregnancy and allow a fertilized egg to implant.

5. Miscarriage chance: If some hormonal imbalances are not effectively handled during pregnancy, such as thyroid issues, the chance of miscarriage may increase.

Effect on Fertility in Men:

1. Low Testosterone: Low testosterone levels can impact male fertility by

causing a drop in sperm production and quality.

2. Erectile Dysfunction: Imbalances in hormones can lead to erectile dysfunction, which affects a man's capacity for both conception and sexual activity.

3. Health of Sperm: Imbalances in hormones can have a detrimental effect on motility and quality of sperm, decreasing the likelihood of conception.

Therapy and Administration:

- Depending on the particular disease, therapeutic options for hormonal imbalances that impair fertility and pregnancy may include hormone replacement therapy, lifestyle changes, medication, and surgical procedures.

In order to improve fertility in women, it can be extremely important to monitor ovulation, treat irregular menstruation, and take care of hormonal abnormalities like PCOS or thyroid issues.

- Improving general health, sexual function, and testosterone abnormalities in males can all improve fertility.

- Assisted reproductive methods such as intrauterine insemination (IUI) or in vitro fertilization (IVF) may be considered if hormonal abnormalities are unresolvable.

Reproductive endocrinologists and fertility experts are among the medical professionals that individuals and couples dealing with fertility issues should consult. The likelihood of a successful pregnancy can be considerably increased by early detection and treatment of hormone abnormalities. Furthermore, the health of the mother and the unborn child depends on prenatal care and careful management of hormonal abnormalities during pregnancy.

B. Taking Care of Your Hormones While Pregnant

The mother's and the developing baby's health during pregnancy depend on managing hormone levels. Significant hormonal changes occur throughout pregnancy, so it's important to keep things in balance for a successful pregnancy. When it comes to regulating hormonal health throughout pregnancy, keep the following points in mind:

1. Maternal Health:

Frequent prenatal visits are necessary to track the developing baby's and the mother's health. Healthcare professionals will measure hormone levels, treat any hormonal issues, and offer advice on maintaining hormonal health throughout these visits.

2. Thyroid Function:

- The functioning of the thyroid is particularly crucial during pregnancy. The development of the baby's brain is greatly influenced by thyroid hormones. It's critical to work with your healthcare professional to make sure your thyroid hormone levels are within the prescribed range if you have a thyroid problem.

3. Control of Blood Sugar:

Blood sugar levels might be affected by pregnancy. In order to effectively manage their blood sugar, women with gestational diabetes or preexisting diabetes must keep an eye on it and collaborate with a healthcare team.

4. Conditions Connected to Hormones:

- Preexisting hormonal disorders, such as hyperprolactinemia or polycystic ovarian syndrome (PCOS), may affect some women. In order to lower potential dangers during pregnancy, proper care and monitoring are essential.

5. Supplemental Hormones:

- To preserve hormonal balance during pregnancy, doctors may occasionally prescribe hormone supplements or other drugs. Progesterone pills, for instance, are occasionally used to assist in the initial phases of pregnancy.

6, Emotional Health:

- Changes in hormones during pregnancy may also have an impact on mood. It's critical to take care of one's mental health and get help for ailments like anxiety and sadness.

7. Diet and Nutrition:

In order to maintain hormonal health throughout pregnancy, a diet rich in nutrients and well-balanced is essential. Make sure you're receiving enough vitamins and minerals to support your growing child as well as yourself.

8. Engaging in Exercise:

Maintaining a healthy weight, controlling hormones, and lowering stress levels can all be achieved with moderate physical activity during pregnancy. For pregnancy-specific exercise suggestions, speak with your healthcare physician.

9: Rest:

Hormonal equilibrium depends on getting a good night's sleep. Improve your sleeping environment and give rest priority because pregnancy can cause discomfort and disrupt sleep.

10. Stay Hydrated

Maintaining proper hydration is crucial for general health and can help maintain hormonal balance.

11. Steer clear of hazardous substances:

Avoid alcohol, tobacco, and recreational drugs as they might cause hormonal imbalances and harm to your unborn child.

12. Stress Reduction:

- Reduce your stress by using methods like deep breathing, mindfulness, and relaxation exercises. This will lessen the negative effects of stress on hormone balance.

13. Nursing a baby:

- After pregnancy, hormonal changes persist during nursing. Hormone levels, particularly those related to milk production, might be impacted by nursing.

It's critical that you and your healthcare practitioner be in constant contact during your pregnancy. They can offer advice on maintaining hormonal health as well as help with any hormonal issues. Individualized treatment and monitoring are essential to guarantee a healthy pregnancy and a safe delivery because every pregnancy is different.

Chapter 11: Mental Health and Hormonal Imbalance

A. Hormones and Emotional Health

Hormones and emotional health are closely related. Hormones are important for controlling mood, feelings, and mental health in general. Knowing this connection can help us better understand how hormonal imbalances affect emotional health and how emotional health affects hormonal balance. Key details concerning this link are as follows:

1. Stress Hormones:

- There is a strong correlation between stress chemicals, especially cortisol, and emotional health. Anxiety, tension, and even melancholy can be attributed to elevated cortisol levels in response to stress.

2. Hormones that Regulate Mood:

- Neurotransmitters that are important for controlling mood include dopamine and serotonin. Anxiety and sadness are two mood disorders that can result from imbalances in these neurotransmitters.

3. Hormonal fluctuations with the menstrual cycle:

- Hormonal fluctuations in women during the menstrual cycle might impact their emotional state and overall mood. The symptoms of premenstrual syndrome (PMS) and premenstrual dysphoric disorder (PMDD) include mood swings linked to hormonal changes.

4. Postpartum and Pregnancy:

- Changes in hormones during and after pregnancy might have an impact on a person's emotional health. During these times, hormones like progesterone and estrogen contribute to mood swings. One example of a mood illness linked to hormonal changes following childbirth is postpartum depression.

5. Hormonal Dysregulation and Mental Health Disorders:

- Mental health issues and mood problems can be exacerbated by hormonal abnormalities, such as those caused by PCOS and thyroid disorders.

6. Hormone Production and Emotional Stress:

- Hormone production and regulation may be impacted by long-term emotional stress. Hormonal imbalances brought on by stress might have an effect on one's emotional well-being.

7. Strategies for Emotional Well-Being:

- Techniques that improve mental health, such as mindfulness, meditation, and yoga, can aid in stress reduction and hormone balance.

8. Hormonal and Physical Well-Being:

- A healthy lifestyle that includes regular exercise, a balanced diet, and enough sleep can have a favorable effect on both hormonal balance and emotional well-being.

9. Expert Assistance

Seek advice from medical professionals if you have ongoing emotional difficulties or believe a hormonal imbalance is influencing your mood. They are able to offer diagnostic evaluations and suggest suitable courses of action.

Physical, mental, and emotional aspects all play a part in the comprehensive process of managing hormonal balance and emotional well-being. Understanding the connection between hormones and emotions emphasizes how crucial it is to treat both in order to improve overall well being.

B. Dealing with Anxiety and Mood Swings

Although managing anxiety and mood swings might be difficult, there are useful tactics and methods that can support you. The following advice will help you manage anxiety and mood swings:

1.Determine Triggers:

- Be mindful of the circumstances or elements that set off your anxiety and mood swings. You can better control and predict your reactions by being aware of this.

2. Inhaling deeply and unwinding:

- To ease tension and quiet your thoughts, try deep breathing exercises and relaxation methods. Particularly useful methods include gradual muscular relaxation.

3. Meditation and Mindfulness:

- Practice mindfulness and meditation to stay in the present moment and lessen the influence of erratic thoughts and moods.

4. Engaging in Exercise:

Frequent exercise can lessen anxiety and elevate mood. Include a hobby or favorite activity in your daily routine, such as yoga, walking, or sports.

5. Rest:

Make good sleep a priority because getting too little sleep can make anxiety and mood swings worse. Establish a calming nighttime routine and stick to a regular sleep schedule.

6. Nutritious Diet:

- Anxiety can be lessened and mood can be improved with a healthy, nutrient-dense diet. Steer clear of sugary foods and excessive coffee intake as these might cause energy spikes and crashes.

7. Maximum Tension: stress

- Control stress by setting priorities, managing your time, and finding practical solutions to problems. Acknowledge when you require pauses and engage in self-care.

8. Expert Assistance:

- You should think about getting expert mental health assistance if anxiety and mood fluctuations are having a big influence on your day-to-day activities. Medication, counseling, or therapy might be useful forms of treatment.

9. Journaling:

- To better understand your emotions and triggers, put your ideas and feelings in writing. Using a journal to communicate and analyze your experiences can be beneficial.

10. Assistance Program:

Seek assistance from friends and relatives. It can be relieving and a way to connect to talk about your feelings with someone you trust.

11. Cognitive-Behavioral Methods:

- Take into consideration cognitive-behavioral therapy (CBT), a methodical and goal-oriented technique that modifies unfavorable thought patterns and behavior patterns to treat anxiety and mood fluctuations.

12. Medication:

- To treat severe anxiety or mood problems, a doctor's prescription may be required in some circumstances.

13. Self-Acceptance:

Treat yourself with patience and kindness. Recognize that everyone goes through periods of anxiety and mood swings, and that it's acceptable to ask for assistance and support when necessary.

14. Restrict Excitation:

- Cut back on or give up stimulants like nicotine and caffeine, as these can make anxiety and mood swings worse.

15. Stick to a Schedule:

- Create a daily schedule that consists of rest, exercise, and regular mealtimes. Structure and predictability can aid in mood stabilization.

16. Breathwork Activities:

- Develop diaphragmatic breathing, which involves taking a deep inhale through your nose and letting it out gradually via your mouth. This may aid in lowering anxiety and calming the neurological system.

Recall that managing anxiety and mood swings is a process, and it's acceptable to get professional assistance if necessary. Maintaining regular self-care, stress reduction, and health-promoting behaviors can have a big impact on your capacity to control these feelings and improve your general wellbeing.

Chapter 12:. Resources and Support

A. Healthcare professionals and experts

Specialists and medical professionals are vital to the healthcare industry because they provide a variety of skills for managing, diagnosing, and treating a wide range of medical disorders.

The following are some important medical experts and specialists:

1. Primary Care Physicians (PCs):

- For individuals seeking medical attention, PCPs are frequently the initial point of contact. They address common health conditions, provide routine check-ups, and offer general medical care.

2. Pediatricians

- Pediatricians focus on treating the distinct medical requirements and developmental milestones of newborns, kids, and teenagers.

3. Internists:

- Internists, or internal medicine physicians, specialize in providing healthcare to adults, identifying and managing a variety of ailments.

4. Family doctors:

- Family doctors act as primary care physicians, offering individuals and families of all ages comprehensive treatment.

5. Gynecologists and obstetricians, or OB/GYNs:

- OB/GYNs are specialists in women's health, including prenatal and obstetric care in addition to treatment for gynecological and reproductive disorders.

6. Cardiologist

- Cardiologists treat disorders pertaining to the cardiovascular system and are specialists in heart health.

7. Skin specialists:

Dermatologists diagnose and treat a wide range of dermatological problems with an emphasis on the health of the skin, hair, and nails.

8. Experts in neurology:

- Neurologists treat diseases like epilepsy, multiple sclerosis, and Parkinson's disease. They are experts in illnesses of the nervous system, which includes the brain and spinal cord.

9. Psychologist:

Medical professionals that specialize in the diagnosis and treatment of mental health conditions such as schizophrenia, bipolar disorder, anxiety, and depression are known as psychiatrists.

10. Orthopedic Physicians:

- Orthopedic surgeons treat diseases of the musculoskeletal system, which includes disorders of the bones, joints, and soft tissues. When surgery is required, they carry it out.

11. Digestive surgeons:

- Treating conditions including Crohn's disease, gastrointestinal malignancies, and irritable bowel syndrome, gastroenterologists concentrate on the digestive system.

12. Eye specialists:

- Ophthalmologists are specialists in the eyes who do surgery on the eyes as well as diagnose and treat eye disorders.

13. Dentists:

- Dentists offer dental treatment, including cleanings, fillings, and oral surgery. They are specialists in oral health.

14. Doctors of urology:

Urologists address ailments like kidney stones and prostate problems, specializing in the male reproductive system and the urinary tract.

15. Pulmonologists

- Pulmonologists treat ailments including asthma, chronic obstructive pulmonary disease (COPD), and sleep apnea with an emphasis on respiratory health.

16.. Immunologists and allergists:

- Immunologists and allergists identify and treat immune system abnormalities and allergic reactions.

17. Diabetologists:

- Diabetes, thyroid issues, and hormonal imbalances are among the illnesses and ailments that endocrinologists specialize in.

18. In rheumatology:

- Rheumatologists treat autoimmune disorders and ailments affecting the connective tissues and joints.

19. Cancer specialists:

Specialists in cancer diagnosis, treatment, and care coordination are known as oncologists.

20. Nephrologists

Diagnosing and treating illnesses and problems connected to the kidneys is the primary focus of nephrologists.

Together, these healthcare providers form a coordinated healthcare system that offers patients comprehensive and specialized care. You may consult with one or more of these specialists to obtain the right diagnosis and course of treatment, depending on your particular medical requirements.

B. Support Communities and Online Groups

For anyone dealing with medical illnesses, needing emotional support, or experiencing health challenges, support groups and online communities can be invaluable resources. These communities offer a feeling of belonging, comprehension, and a forum for knowledge and experience exchange. Here are a few instances of online communities and support groups:

1. Local Support Groups:

These are frequently arranged by nonprofits, community centers, or medical clinics. They make it possible for people dealing with related health problems to get together in person and exchange stories.

2. Forums for Online Health:

- A lot of websites and social media platforms feature health forums and discussion groups where users may ask questions, exchange personal experiences, and get in touch with others dealing with related health issues. MedHelp, PatientsLikeMe, and HealthBoards are a few examples.

3. Particular Groups Based on Conditions:

- Online forums and support groups catering to particular medical disorders exist. For instance, there are communities for multiple sclerosis, diabetes support groups, and cancer patients.

4. Help for Mental Health:

- People can talk about mental health concerns and get help in online groups like 7 Cups, Psych Central, and Reddit's mental health subreddits.

5. Groups for parents and caregivers:

- Whether they are looking after elderly family members or youngsters with special needs, parents and caregivers frequently look for help in communities where they can interact with others who are in similar situations.

6. Orphan Conditions and Rare Diseases:

There are devoted online forums for a number of rare diseases where patients and their families can interact with others who have similar experiences and obtain information.

7. Communities for Women's Health:

- Women's health issues, such as those pertaining to menopause, infertility, pregnancy, and gynecological disorders, are the subject of internet forums.

8. LGBTQ+ Health Assistance:

- Online groups can offer a secure setting where LGBTQ+ people can talk about particular health issues, exchange stories, and look for advice.

9. Chronic Pain Assistance:

- People who have chronic pain can locate online support groups that provide guidance, tools, and emotional support for dealing with pain and associated ailments.

10. Groups for general health and wellness:

Certain communities prioritize the advancement of overall health and well-being by means of talks about stress management, fitness, diet, and lifestyle modifications.

11. Instagram Groups:

- There are numerous Facebook groups devoted to health issues, encompassing a broad spectrum of ailments and passions. These groups facilitate conversation, the exchange of advice, and support.

12. Online Resources for Counseling:

- Certain platforms offer a more discreet and expert form of help by connecting users with qualified therapists and counselors via chat, phone conversations, or video calls.

The following should be kept in mind when engaging in online communities and support groups:

- Honor others' confidentiality and privacy.

- Look for guidance and information based on evidence, particularly when talking about medical issues or therapies.

- Recognize that not all internet information is trustworthy or truthful.

- Use these communities in addition to, not as a substitute for, expert medical guidance and care.

Making connections with others who are sympathetic to your predicament can be incredibly enlightening, emotionally supportive, and less isolating. To receive individualized medical advice and care, you should, nevertheless, always speak with a healthcare provider.

C. Additional Reading and Sources

Here are some resources to take into consideration if you're looking for additional reading and references on any of the subjects covered or on any particular medical disorders or treatments:

1. Medical Databases and Journals:

- A complete database of papers and articles related to medical research is available at PubMed (pubmed.ncbi.nlm.nih.gov).

-Reputable medical periodicals are The New England Journal of Medicine and JAMA (Journal of the American Medical Association).

-A search engine for scholarly articles is Google Scholar (scholar.google.com).

2. Books:

Seek out publications authored by specialists and medical professionals to gain comprehensive knowledge on particular subjects. The highly regarded medical reference book "The Merck Manual of Diagnosis and Therapy" is one example.

3. Agencies for Government Health:

Sites such as the U.S. Reputable sources of health information are the Centers for Disease Control and Prevention (CDC) at cdc.gov and the National Institutes of Health (NIH) at nih.gov.

4. Associations for Medicine:

- Look for information about particular medical specialties by visiting the websites of medical associations like the American Medical Association (ama-assn.org) or the American Heart Association (heart.org).

5. Web-based Health Resources:

- There are a plethora of information and resources available on a variety of health topics on websites such as WebMD (webmd.com), Mayo Clinic (mayoclinic.org), and Healthline (healthline.com).

6. College Health Centers:

- Reputable university medical facilities' websites frequently offer trustworthy information about health and medical research. The Cleveland Clinic (my.clevelandclinic.org) and the Mayo Clinic (mayoclinic.org) are two examples.

7. Educational Establishments:

- Look through university and academic institution websites for scholarly publications and research papers on particular medical topics.

8. Departments of Health in Government:

- Public health and specialty publications are frequently released by the health authorities in your nation or area.

9. Advocacy groups for patients:

- A plethora of patient advocacy groups and foundations focused on certain medical illnesses offer resources, support, and information.

-The Alzheimer's Association (alz.org) and the American Cancer Society (cancer.org) are two examples.

10. Healthcare News Sources:

- Visit reliable news sites like MedPage Today (medpage.com) and Medscape (medscape.com) to stay up to current on medical news.

11. Medical Service Providers:

Asking your healthcare physician for recommended reading materials related to your illness or concerns is never a bad idea.

Consider seriously evaluating the sources you use, and make sure the data is accurate and supported by proof. For specific medical advice and direction catered to your particular set of medical requirements, always seek the assistance of a healthcare professional.

Conclusion

A. Recap of Key Takeaways

The following summarizes the main conclusions from our conversation on several health and wellness-related topics:

The Function of Hormones in the Body:

-Hormones are chemical messengers that control metabolism, development, and reproduction, among other body processes.

-Hormones are produced and released by major glands, including the pituitary, thyroid, and adrenal glands.

The balance of hormones is essential for general health and wellbeing.

Typical Reasons for Hormonal Disproportion:

-Hormonal imbalances can be caused by a number of things, including drugs, aging, stress, and medical disorders.

- Lifestyle decisions about food, exercise, and sleep affect hormonal health.
- A variety of symptoms and health problems can be brought on by hormonal imbalances.

Identifying Signs and Symptoms:

-Hormonal imbalance symptoms might vary, but they can include mood swings, exhaustion, weight fluctuations, and irregular menstruation cycles.

-It's critical to recognize these signs and, if required, seek medical attention.

Medical Assessment and Diagnosis:

-Healthcare practitioners can use blood testing and other diagnostic techniques to identify hormonal abnormalities.

- Treating and managing patients effectively requires an accurate diagnosis.

Getting Expert Assistance:

-Seek advice and therapy from endocrinologists or other professionals regarding hormone abnormalities.

-Maintaining good health management requires open communication with your healthcare team.

Diet and Nutrition:

- Hormone health is supported by a diet rich in nutrients and balanced with meals.

- Vitamins, minerals, and omega-3 fatty acids are nutrients that are crucial for maintaining hormonal equilibrium.

Steer clear of processed foods and excessive sugar as they may interfere with hormone function.

Movement and Physical Exercise:

Frequent exercise, such as aerobic and weight training, supports hormonal equilibrium.

- Exercise lowers the chance of hormone abnormalities and helps manage stress.

Stress Reduction:

Prolonged stress can harm one's health by causing hormonal abnormalities.

- Stress-reduction methods including mindfulness, meditation, and deep breathing exercises might be beneficial.

Hormone Reactions to Sleep:

- Immune system performance, hormone balance, and general health all depend on getting enough sleep.

- Creating a cozy sleeping environment and sticking to a regular sleep routine might enhance the quality of your sleep.

Herbal supplements and natural remedies:

- Seek medical advice before taking any supplements or natural therapies.

Treatment with Hormone Replacement (HRT):

- One medical intervention for hormonal abnormalities is hormone replacement therapy.

- It entails substituting synthetic or bioidentical hormones for hormones that are lacking.

Alternative Medicine (Yoga, Acupuncture, etc.):

- Complementing conventional treatments, alternative therapies like aromatherapy, yoga, and acupuncture can support hormonal balance.

Rich in Nutrients Foods:

- Nutrient-rich foods, such as fruits, vegetables, whole grains, and lean meats, improve hormonal balance and general wellness.

Hormone-Supportive Dietary Strategies:

- Whole foods are the focus of diets like the DASH and Mediterranean, which can improve hormonal balance.

The Value of Consistent Physical Activity

- Hormone balance, weight control, and general health all depend on regular physical activity.

Exercises for Hormone Regulation Types:

- Strength training, flexibility training, and aerobic exercise combined can support hormone regulation.

Meditation & Mindfulness:

- Meditation and mindfulness techniques help lower stress, enhance mental health, and support hormonal balance.

Calming Activities:

- Stress management and relaxation can be facilitated by methods such as progressive muscle relaxation, guided imagery, and deep breathing.

Reducing Stress in Everyday Life:

Hormonal health depends on stress management techniques such as time management, priority setting, and self-care.

The Value of Good Sleep

- Adequate sleep is essential for hormonal equilibrium, mental clarity, and general well-being.

Suitable Sleep Positions:

Improving sleep quality can be achieved by keeping a regular sleep schedule and designing a sleep-friendly atmosphere.

Hormonal Unbalance during Various Phases of Life:

Hormonal imbalances can arise during different phases of life, including but not limited to puberty, reproductive years, pregnancy, menopause, and aging.

Effects on Pregnancy and Fertility:

- Pregnancy and fertility can be impacted by hormonal abnormalities. For positive results, proper administration and care are necessary.

Taking Care of Your Hormones While Pregnant:

-Hormone health during pregnancy is mostly dependent on lifestyle decisions, prenatal care, and hormone monitoring.

Hormones and Emotional Wellness:

- The regulation of mood and emotions is greatly influenced by hormones. It is crucial to comprehend this relationship in order to manage emotional wellness.

Handling Anxiety and Mood Swings:

-Coping mechanisms for anxiety and mood swings include recognizing stressors, using relaxation methods, getting support from a professional, and leading a healthy lifestyle.

Specialists and Practitioners in Medicine:

- Healthcare services are provided for certain medical requirements by a variety of medical professionals and specialists, such as surgeons, specialists, and primary care physicians.

Support Communities and Online Groups:

- For people dealing with health issues, support groups and online communities provide a network of connections, emotional support, and information exchange.

Additional Readings and Sources:

For in-depth information on certain health topics, consult academic institutions, government health organizations, medical associations, books, medical journals, and internet sites.

A wide range of subjects pertaining to wellbeing, hormone balance, and health are covered in these key takeaways. It is advisable to get advice and guidance from healthcare professionals specifically tailored to your individual health needs.

In summary, a key element of general wellbeing for both men and women is hormonal health. Leading a healthy and satisfying life requires knowing the role of hormones, spotting the warning signs of hormonal imbalances, and taking proactive measures to control hormonal health.

We covered a wide range of subjects in our conversation, from the fundamentals of hormones and typical causes of hormonal imbalances to the significance of lifestyle choices like sleep, stress reduction, exercise, and diet in preserving hormonal balance. We also talked about the importance of mental health, how to manage anxiety and mood swings, and how support networks and medical professionals can offer direction and assistance.

It's critical to keep in mind that each person's journey toward optimal hormonal health is distinct. Hormonal balance may be enjoyed by some, while others may experience difficulties. In order to promote and sustain hormonal health, regardless of your circumstances, education, awareness, and proactive self-care are essential.

People can take charge of their hormonal health by connecting with support networks, remaining informed, and seeking expert assistance when necessary. Women and men alike can improve their general quality of life and well-being by making educated decisions, embracing healthy lifestyles, and taking care of hormone difficulties.

Recall that maintaining hormonal balance is essential to a more comprehensive strategy for holistic health. Making self-care a priority, going to the doctor on a regular basis, and adopting healthy habits can all lead to a balanced and satisfying existence.

You are actively working toward a healthier and happier you by implementing the suggestions covered

in this talk. Your health and well-being
are worth the effort.